I've got Something to Say

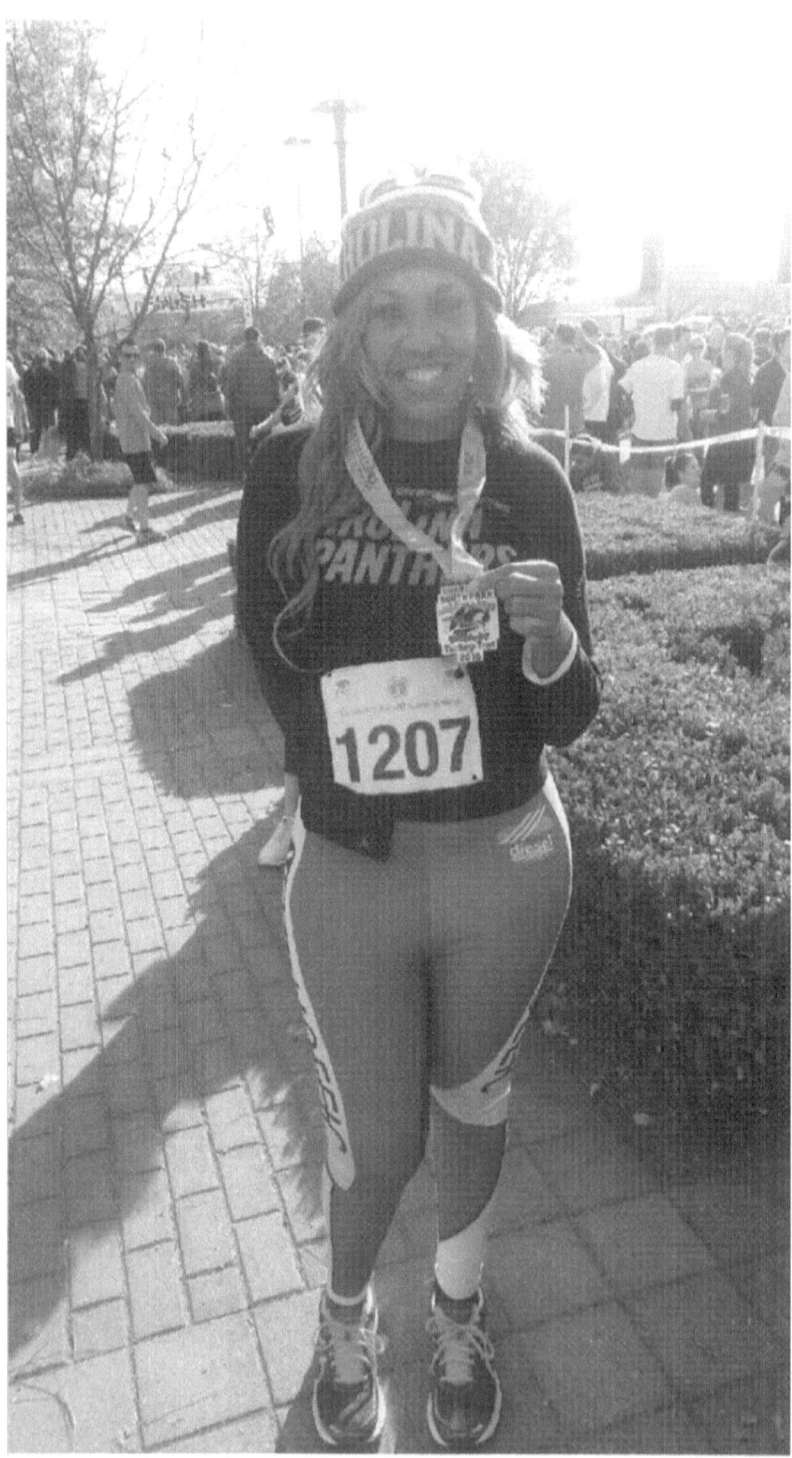

I've got Something to Say

My Weight loss Journey

Dr. Dee Honeycutt

ISBN: 978-1-365-89583-8

To order additional copies of this book, contact:
drdeehoneycutt@gmail.com

Dedication

I would like to thank God because none of this would be possible without him. He blessed me with wisdom, patience and discipline.

I want to say thank you to (Apostle Ann Decoteau) for continually keeping me in her prayers. You always help me with spiritual guidance but at the same time you always keep it real and never judge me, so thank you for that.

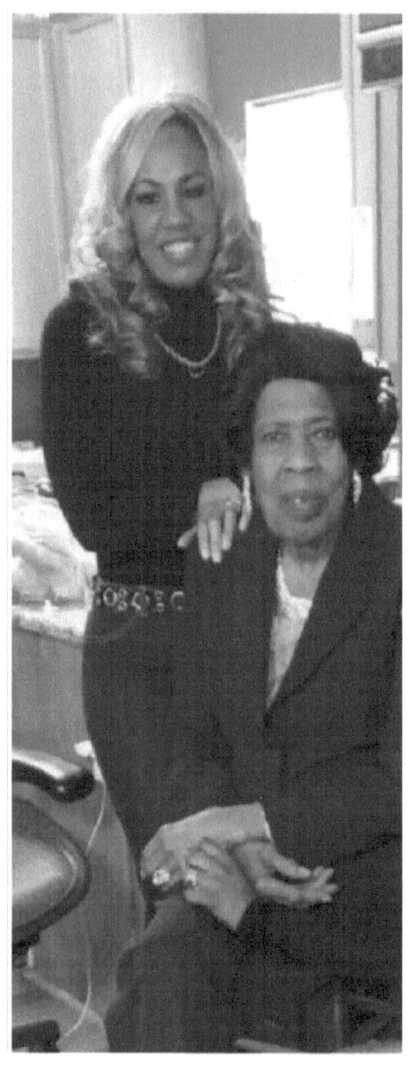

I love this lady she is the backbone of my success. My dear mom, Evelyn Davis

Table of Contents

Acknowledgements 8

About thebook...9

An honest conversation with your body 10

About Me...12

Is water really that important to ourdiets?......................22

What is Candida? 24

Vitamins and Supplements...28

Garlic 31

Liver Health...32

Benefits of Exercise 34

Conclusion 42

MealPlans..44

Acknowledgements

Special thanks to my golden girls you all have always believed in me and support everything I do.

Andrea Newman DeAndrea Newman Jimmie Chaplain-Wilkerson My friends and family

Gi Gi Springs you always said if I said it's was gonna happen it's done. Last but not least an extra special thanks to my mom she has always been my number one fan.

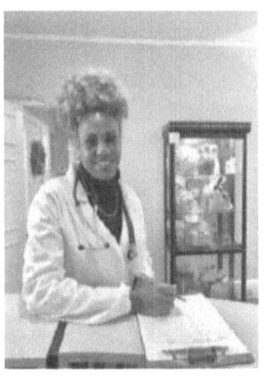

About the book

This is a book to expand health and wellness awareness in the community. More and more health care professionals are professing the importance of preventive measures as the makeup of a healthy future, which decreases health care cost stremendously.

This book is a manual in which I will focus on the experience I have had being overweight; a struggle which led to my passion to learn to live a healthy life and ultimately receive a Bachelor of Arts (B.A.) in Nutrition. While designed to let you know that others have weight loss challenges and you are not alone within the endeavor to lose weight and maintain a healthy life, please note that the meal plans detailed in this book are only suggestions. You are advised to seek guidance from your medical doctor for clearance before using the guide. As you go through the guide, please write down your goals to change your lifestyle to a newer and healthier you. Once you have finished, please apply the best practices you have captured, as what you write will assist you in meeting your goals. Now, let's get started!

An honest conversation with your body

If your body could talk what would it say...
Would it say that you are healthy, fit or out of shape, or
would it say that you are carrying too much weight.

Are you giving it enough water to drink, do you give it
enough time to sleep, do you give it the right foods to
eat,
Are your lungs suffocating from smoke and is liver
drowning in alcohol?

Look in the mirror and ask yourself these questions,
How do you think that your body would respond to
these questions?

Making healthy choices can add years to your life, and Yes
there will be things that you will have to sacrifice,
Like giving up fried foods and eating desserts at
midnight.

A positive change would be worth it, progress towards the
future, So that your body can say,
"Thank you for taking care of me and I shall remain healthy."

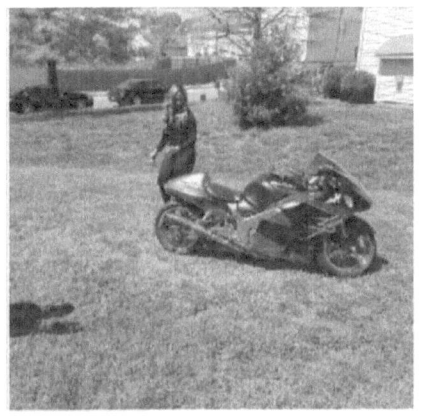

Written by: DeShaunda Honeycutt

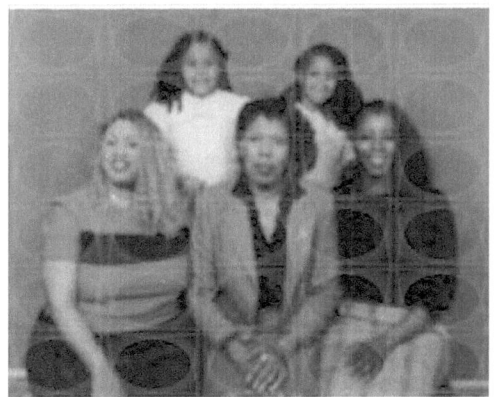

About Me

While studying to receive my Bachelors in Holistic nutrition and Doctorate in Naturopathy, I discovered that I have a gift from God to help people learn to live a healthy lifestyle. My goal is to reach people of all races; regardless if they are skinny, fat, young, or old; sickness and obesity does not discriminate. I have had a weight challenge all my life but I found my body's secret to maintain my weight and you can too.

My familial history, both maternal and paternal, includes a history of hypertension and diabetes. This is a primary reason that I will watch my food choices every day of my life. This was not always my viewpoint. The phrase, "you are what you eat", is very true. If you eat junk and fatty foods you will feel that way. I will not claim to have all of the answers or a quick fix but I have learned a lot from the actual experience of being overweight. One of the keys to successful weight loss is to make a lifestyle change that includes a healthy diet; something we have heard time and time again. Keeping a food diary is very important, as well. I tell my patients to write down everything they eat, which includes the good, bad, or ugly.

Thinking back, I remember the highest weight in my life; I was tipping the scales at a whopping 238 pounds! At each doctor visit, my blood pressure would read borderline high. I had enough sense to know that I was on the road to destruction; first hypertension then diabetes and high cholesterol that could one day lead to a heart attack or stroke.

I always felt sluggish and my self-esteem was extremely low. I remember a conversation that my cousin and I had about losing weight. My cousin said that she wanted to lose weight so bad that she wished she would get sick with something that would make her shed the pounds. That was not a good thought, was it? Another time, I remember turning to a doctor to receive diet pills. Sure enough, I lost 25 pounds in a month.

When I started eating again, I gained those 25 pounds back plus a whole lot more, at the height of my struggles, there was a diet clinic that came through Charlotte. At that time, I saw that as my hope, as I had the opportunity to receive daily support to achieve results. I lost more than 80 pounds in six months but what the clinic did not know is that I was barely eating anything at all.

If I had known then what I know now, I should have been eating healthy small quantities of food throughout the day and the weight would have come off quicker than it actually did—and stayed off. I kept a good bit of that weight off. I never made it back to 238 pounds but I did see 199 for many years. I thought that weighing 199 was okay because I became comfortable not hearing the word fat, (you know that is the first thing that a person looks for when they see you). They cant wait to comment; "You're gaining that weight back arent you". Not "Oh girl, it is so good to see you". Society can be the pits sometimes.

In 2004, I went to my doctor and I asked her why she thought I was having such an issue losing weight. Again, she asked me some questions and told me to try a few things. Before I left, the last thing that she told me was if those things didnt help me, she would check my thyroid gland the following year when I came for my physical. I dont know about you, but when a doctor tells me that she wants to run a test to check my thyroid, a little light came on to get it together and keep it together.

When a good doctor advises you that your glucose level is high or you have high blood pressure, their primary advice will request that you change your diet and walk. They might suggest that you increase your cardio and come back to have your levels checked again to determine if the introduction of those things into you daily life will save and extend your life, while improving your overall health. I intentionally made mention of a 'good' doctor, because doctors who are not so good will not hesitate to put you on medication the very first time your levels are high, so do not make the mistake of waiting until your body is headed for destruction to make positive changes. Why not make a lifestyle change that could prevent negative impacts to your health and add healthy years to your life? I pray this book will inspire those who think that they cannot make a lifestyle change. As people are reading about my personal plight, I pray they will find it within themselves to keep going and remember that I was them at one point in my life. I am not trying to write a story about my life but the reality is that weight has always been a very big part of my life.

I 2005,I embarked upon a total lifestyle change, in which included earning a BA in Holistic Nutrition Studies, which afforded me the credentials and expertise necessary to consult patients on how to lose weight in a healthy manner. This also allowed me to lead by example, become a role model, and command charge of my own life, first. I couldnt be overweight and give someone health advice on how to lose weight. Dont get me wrong I am not a size zero. Guess what? I dont have any desire to be a size zero. I am comfortable in my skin and my levels are great. If I was still obese or fat like I was in the past I would receive no respect, people would look at me with the mental question, "Why arent you on your own plan?" In reality, I wouldnt take advice from an overweight doctor or an overweight, weight loss practitioner.

That would be no different than a doctor, who tells a person to stop smoking because it will give you cancer if you dont stop then the doctor lights up a cigar during your consultation. I am not trying to say that losing weight is an easy task because it is not. If you achieve an understanding about how the body works along with breaking down food, it will open up a whole new ball game in the healthy weight loss world. This is why I am so compelled to write this book and in the near future I will record some motivational CDs. I cant tell you anything about being a drug addict or an alcoholic but I can definitely relate to having an addiction to food. In other words, just like a person that has an eating disorder, binge eats or just makes wrong food choices that they know affects their weight, destiny is controlled by the decisions that we make not our situations. We truly have to rehabilitate our thinking patterns toward our food and our bodies. I am a faithful believer that God has equipped us with everything that we need to be healthy individuals but we have to reform mentally and physically to use the abilities that we have.

Your blood sugar plays a very important factor in healthy weight loss. If your blood sugar is not balanced you will experience low energy levels and consequently weight issues. You see the level of glucose in our blood has a large responsibility in relation to our appetite. We feel hungry when the level drops. I know sometimes it seems like sweets are calling our names. Right? As human beings we are attracted to the way carbohydrates taste. Specifically we love the sweetness in the goodies that we eat but goodies usually contain one of the many forms of sugar. The forms of sugar are white and brown sugar, honey, glucose, and a few more forms of sugars, which are all fast releasing and cause a really fast increase in the blood sugar levels. When our bodies cannot use the sugar, it is put into storage and eventually turns into fat. Have you ever noticed how bad you feel after the fact when you go on sugar binges? I know I remember. Ninety-percent of vitamins and minerals are removed from white sugar. If we dont have minerals and vitamins, we experience inefficient metabolism leading to bad energy and terrible weight controls.

Another thing you have to watch is your fruit or should I say watch your choices of fruit. All of the fruit that starts with the letter P are natural laxatives. Fruit contains fructose which is considered a simple sugar that enters the blood stream quickly because it does not need to be digested. Our bodies cant use fructose in its current form. Our cells run on glucose only. In order for our body to use fructose, our body has to convert the fructose into glucose. Guess what? The conversion slows the affect that sugar has on the metabolism. Fruits that are slow releasing are better choices if we are trying to lose weight. Apples are an example of a slow releasing fruit because it is mainly made of fructose. Have you paid attention to most diets that are written? The diets do not recommend bananas, which are high in potassium, in addition; they contain fructose and glucose so they raise blood sugar at a speedy pace. Now you see why I said that first you need education and rehabilitation to successfully achieve a healthy life style change. If you can keep your blood sugar levels controlled you will experience balanced weight and constant good energy. Although my age is not important and not a topic that I plan to discuss, I feel better than I felt when I was 20 years old. My personal opinion is that the glycemic index is important because it determines whether the carbohydrates are slow releasing or fast releasing. You do not have to totally stop eating everything you like because we are human and our bodies have been designed for deviations sometimes. Nevertheless we cant splurge day after day or it will start to take a toll on your body. You also have to keep your goodies in moderation. Plan your day thinking about your meals. If you know that you are going to eat out with a friend or have a luncheon at work, or whatever the case, you should consider walking 15 minutes extra that day to burn some extra calories. I always hear one of my patients make the comment, "I would rather need to lose five pounds than to need to lose40 pounds". I feel the same way. You see I know how fat feels. If you are one of those ladies that believes big is beautiful; kudos to you. I take my hat off to you because big and sexy is one thing but you definitely want to be big, sexy, beautiful and healthy. I was big, beautiful and sexy but my health was moving towards unhealthy. When I was heavier, people would always make the comment, "You are heavy but you have a pretty face". I want my face to go with my body. Let me stress to you one more time I am not a size zero but I am comfortable in my skin. I can walk with my head up. When I was heavy, I knew that I needed to lose weight because of my health. I really think that if I had made a choice to remain fat that society would have made me change because this world is so stereotyped. I need to be healthy because not only am I a doctor but I am also a licensed massage therapist. For 10 years I have utilized my hands to provide massage therapy to many people every week. Many people that I treat are not healthy; people come to me when they are sick to make them feel better. As a result, my immune system has to be strong.

There are so many advantages to a healthy lifestyle change. For instance before I started all this healthy stuff I had chronic sinus problems. Many people can vouch for the benefits of a healthy lifestyle. For the last two years I have had a couple of issues that I'm pretty sure were created because I was in a tight spot filled with cigarette smoke but I still didnt get a sinus infection. I'm telling you that I would have taken antibiotics by now. I am so blessed. A lot of people dont know that some foods can cause sinus and allergy problems. That's why it is good to keep a journal of the foods that you eat daily to determine what elevates your weight or may cause other problems due to certain food groups you may have in your diet. Some people may think they cant live without refined sugars and food choices that lead to a poor diet but if you can wean yourself off of them your body will stop craving them. It is like being addict of some sort because the more you eat the more your body will want. As I stated before, it is very important to keep a journal of everything you eat, which includes the good, the bad and the ugly. You also want to keep a journal of your emotions to keep you in tune with whether you are feeding your emotions on certain days. Always remember if there is a health problem evolving, your diet is a primary healing tool to go to. A healthy diet changes a person's immune response to disease. Dont wait until a red light appears to step up and take control of your life. Good health is a lifestyle process. It is a shame that many medical schools dont teach a lot about prevention of disease. Good nutrition is a very important part of maintaining a healthy life while including exercise for the prevention of disease. The major weapon against disease is improving diet.

I am a believer because every time I had my physical exam, I had border line results for hypertension and cholesterol. Without a shadow of a doubt, I believe I would have developed heart disease by now. After the death of my dad I stopped eating beef and pork. I thought I could never give up hamburgers because they were the best to me at that time. One of the reasons I stopped eating red meat ,our bodies struggle to digest red meat; in addition; it takes three days to digest red meat in our system. People always ask about red meat so now you know. Red meat, which is a highly concentrated protein, can create toxicity in the kidney and form kidney stones.

When you cook red meat, acids are formed in the body. If it is cooked too well done, it creates chemical compounds that could be responsible for causing many diseases such as heart disease, stroke, and cancer according to some scientific studies. These are just some of the things that I have learned about beef but I wasn't aware of before I started my studies.

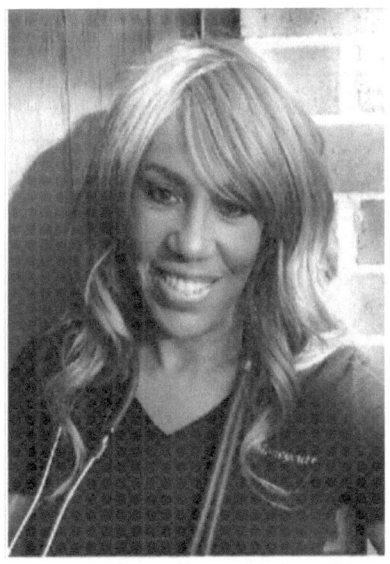

I am so glad that I made that healthy lifestyle change now I can help others improve their daily health one day at a time.

Is water really that important to our diets?

Without water your body breaks down really fast. Every cell that's in the body is regulated and dependent on the correct balance of water. Water is responsible for maintaining body balance, flushing toxins and keeping moisture in the skin. Your bodies use a great deal of water every day through sweating, crying and elimination of urine from your kidneys. Water helps to keep water retention out of the body. Water is a very important tool when it comes to weight loss because it suppresses the appetite naturally and gives you a real feeling of fullness. Not drinking enough water can cause fat deposits to increase. Larger people require more water because of a larger metabolic load and water assists our body in metabolizing stored fat.

Your body excretes about 2 to 3 quarts of water a day. You have to make sure that water is replaced by drinking water so you wont get dehydrated. Water is the only substance that removes fat from the body. According to different research studies a person shouldn't drink water with their meals because it could interfere with absorption of the minerals and vitamins from your foods. Water should be consumed 30 minutes before a meal or 30 minutes after a meal. I prefer that my clients drink a glass of water 30 minutes before their meals so they will have a feeling of fullness, which will help them not over eat and still feel satisfied.

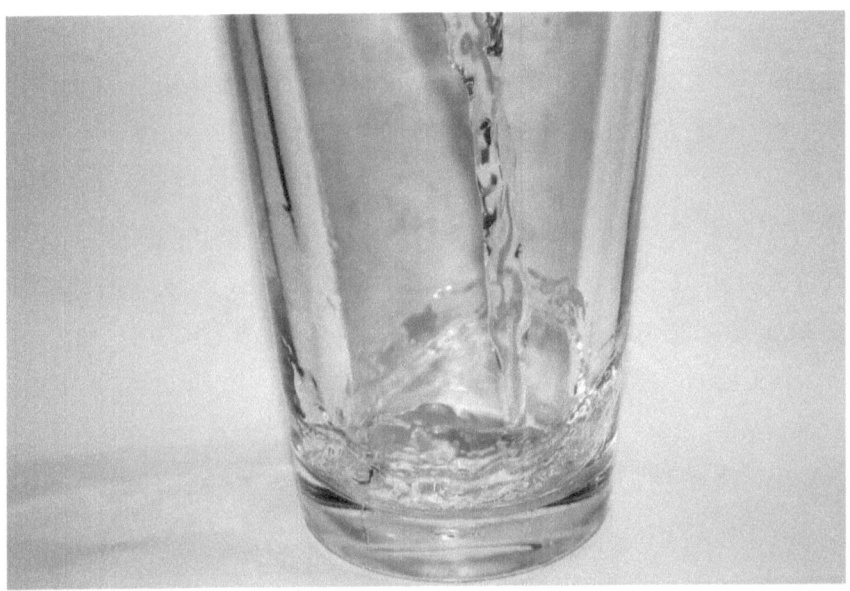

credits by freedigitalphotos.net

What is Candida?

Candida yeast is an imperfect fungi that can be present on the skin in the mucous membranes of the mouth, intestinal tract and vagina that may become pathogenic and eventually cause disease. Candida can also cause thrush and other infections in the body. Many people suffer with Candida overgrowth also known as yeast. It has been stated that one third of all western industrialized countries are affected by this epidemic due to repeated use of antibiotics, steroids as well as a poor diet. According to research, 80 million people suffer from Candida. There are also people living with Candida that have no symptoms. It was brought to my attention while studying for my doctorate how dangerous yeast is to the human body.

I always tell my clients that it grows in our warm dark bodies just like we bake bread in our warm ovens the heat makes the bread rise. There is a strain of Candida called Candida albicans, which is usually a peaceful yeast-like organism that exists in a very limited amount in our digestive tracts from our mouth to our rectum. As long as our immune systems are functioning properly this yeast is kept in check. Candida albicans is a harmless parasite. If the balance of the body's good bacteria is decreased, the immune system is weakened. As a result Candida albicans changes from yeast to a fungus and begins to invade the entire body. The infection is called Candidiasis. The fungus causes a weakening of the cellular structure of our bodies. It is very important to me to make you aware of Candida albicans and Candidiasis.

I am here to tell you that you can be healed from a yeast infection but you have to eat well. The rebalancing of your body chemistry with food will strengthen your immune system and your body tissue will heal. Candida is not just an adult problem; it is a concern for children, teenagers and infants as well. Americans take a great deal of antibiotics, which can have an effect on the whole body system. Antibiotics are usually prescribed for bacterial infections. At that time good and bad bacteria are destroyed causing Candida. Depending on the individual, symptoms may vary from person to person. You would not believe some of the problems that may occur from the association of yeast. Fatigue, problems focusing, memory shortage, joint pain, achy muscles, neck and shoulder tightness, acid reflux, restless sleep, chronic sinusitis, white coated tongue, headaches including migraines, light sensitivity, mood swings, depression, constipation or diarrhea, painful gas and bloating, chills, ear aches allergies, anemia, menstrual problems are only a few of the symptoms but there are many more. Candida is over looked because people dont even think about yeast growing in the body. I decided to include a chapter on Candida in my book to make others aware of what I have learned about the harmful effects of yeast in our bodies. My sister is a daycare owner. When we have spoken I told her that it should be recommended that every child in school or daycare should have a cup of yogurt a day just to keep yeast from turning into a harmful stage. The yogurt will keep a balance of good bacteria in the body. My sister's biggest concern was getting the kids to eat it. Believe me I wish there was a way to ensure that they would eat it. Candida infections are especially prevalent in kids that are prone to infections and require antibiotics; this is true for adults as well. There are lifestyle factors that can be responsible for Candida infections. Some of the factors, which I stated earlier, are repetitive use of antibiotics, poor diet that includes a lot of sugar goods such as starchy breads made with excessive yeast and foods with a lot of chemicals.

We all know that living a high stress life is not good for anyone so that would be a factor too. Yeast can also be aggravated by food allergies. The good news is Candida can be control with changing your diet, keeping sugar to a bare minimum, avoiding antibiotics, birth control, alcohol and tobacco if at all possible. As I stated earlier, yogurt helps keep good bacteria in the tract of the intestines. Garlic is an old time remedy that is best when eaten raw. Women can also use it as a suppository for the vagina. I have a new found love for garlic that I didnt realize until my studies. I preach garlic, garlic, garlic. I will discuss it more in the next chapter entitled, "Vitamins and supplements".

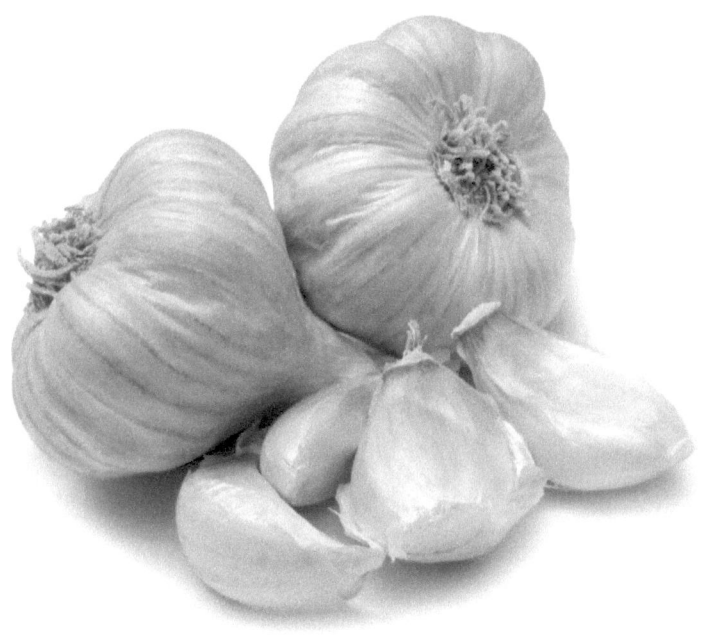

credits by freedigitalphotos.net

Vitamins and Supplements

As I started writing about supplements I looked up at my TV to see six bottles of vitamins. I know that it sounds a little over the top but I am not on any medications. Remember everything is not for everybody. I take a store brand wholesome food multivitamin, fiber capsules, a Candida cleanse, garlic, essential fatty acids, and a supplement for liver health. Now I will discuss each individual vitamin for you. Multivitamins provide hormone balance, strengthen the immune system, enhance healthy skin and supply energy. You can also get the vitamins that you need in your dark leafy and root vegetables, fresh fruit, nuts, and seeds. The multivitamins that I take also have minerals included to enhance every process of the body.

Minerals have many key roles that are responsible for our health. Fiber is very important for preventing constipation. I remember when I was constipated all the time. The only way I would go to the bathroom was to take a laxative. The reason was my poor diet and not enough fiber and water in my diet but now all of that has changed. Sometimes I go to the bathroom even two or three times a day.

Essential fatty acids have many benefits like reducing heart disease, PMS, arthritis, and cancer just to name a few. Omega 6 helps lower blood pressure, improves immune functions, helps balance blood sugar, while Omega 3 keeps cholesterol under control and improves metabolism. There are more essential fatty acids but I wanted you to realize that your doctors are suggesting them to most of their patients. The Candida cleanser is good for healthy digestion which in turn maintains your immune system, which helps to keep infections away. Refer back to my section on Candida because many people dont know that this even occurs in their bodies. You can take probiotics or eat yogurt to get the same benefits as my Candida Cleanser. There are many different types of vitamins to choose from always consult your practitioner before starting a new weight loss program . Everything is not for everyone, the one thing that may work for me could work totally different for you .So invest the best healthy lifestyle change that work for you and watch your life change .Those numbers that was once high when you go get your physical will start to come down and you doctor is going to start asking you questions. I can guarantee you that and the next thing that will come out of his or her mouth is to keep doing what you are doing because it is putting years on to your life.

Fat soluble and water soluble vitamins are two types of major vitamins. Water soluble vitamins such as (B1, B2, B6, and B12), folic acid, niacin and others are not stored within the body because the body is 60% fluid. These vitamins should be consumed daily. Fat soluble vitamins, such as, A, D, E, and K, are responsible for storage and transportation of fat in lipid molecules. One thing I didnt mention when I was talking about minerals is that too many minerals can be toxic to the body.

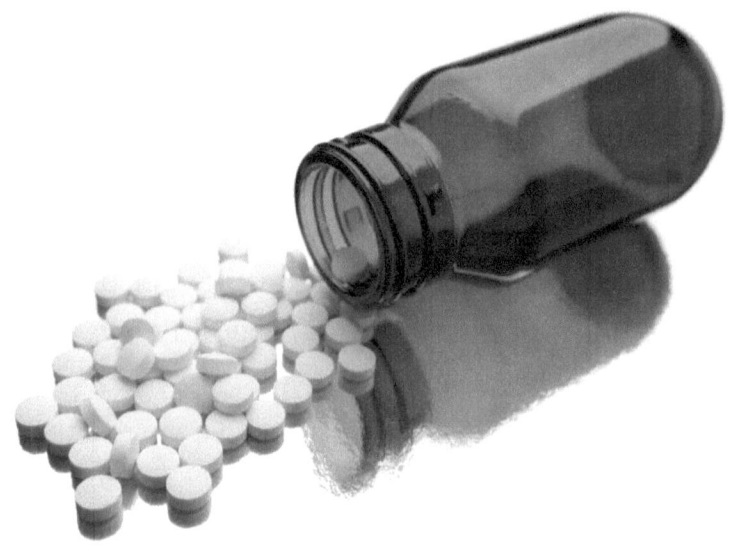

credits by freedigitalphotos.net

Garlic

Garlic is a powerful healing food that has been around for a longtime. There are many good benefits to garlic; it is a natural antibiotic that lowers the risk of colds, helps treat fungal problems and raises the good cholesterol (HDL). There are many more good benefits but I wanted to list the benefits that I think are most important. If you are concerned about the smell of garlic, use the odorless garlic. It took my body a couple of weeks to acclimate to the garlic but now I cant even tell when I have taken it. Any of these supplements that you are interested in starting please consult your physicians before you start them.

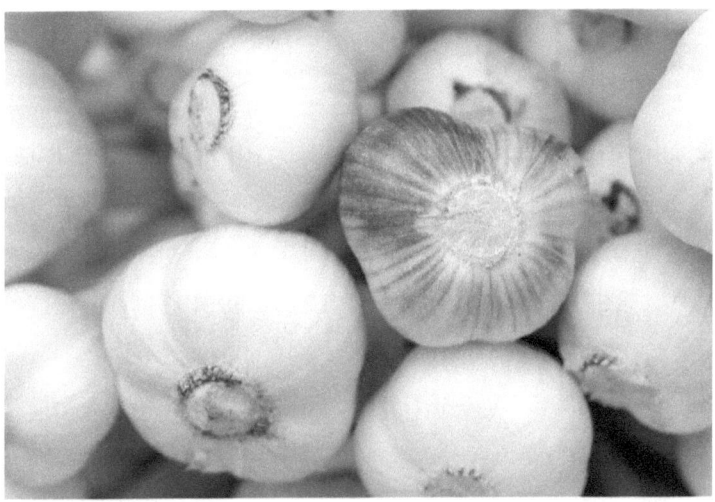

credits by freedigitalphotos.net

Liver Health

Liver health is very important because the liver is the largest organ in our bodies. The liver has many different jobs, it works twenty-four hours a day to keep our blood free from unwanted chemicals, toxins, bacteria's, and other intruders that try to come in and steal good health from the body. The top role of the liver is the detoxification process. Some of the many jobs of the liver include: processing carbohydrates, fats and proteins; storing vitamins and minerals; making or producing bile; detoxifying toxins and filtering the blood to remove poisonous material. A healthy liver should produce a quart of bile a day to eliminate toxins from the body through the bile. If you dont have enough fiber in your body, the bile and toxins may remain in the intestines for a longer period.

If the bile and toxins continue to remain in the intestine and they are not flushed daily, there is the potential for future chronic problems even disease. Your liver is like a filter that keeps out all unwanted guests. In other words it performs a very important job to protect us so we should protect it by eating a proper diet filled with green leafy vegetables as well as increase our water and fiber. There are supplements that work for me but we may take a totally different approach for someone else. It just depends on the individual. I would suggest that everyone take a multivitamin or multi-mineral supplement that your body doesn't absorb from your healthy food choices but consult your own physician or wellness practitioner first.

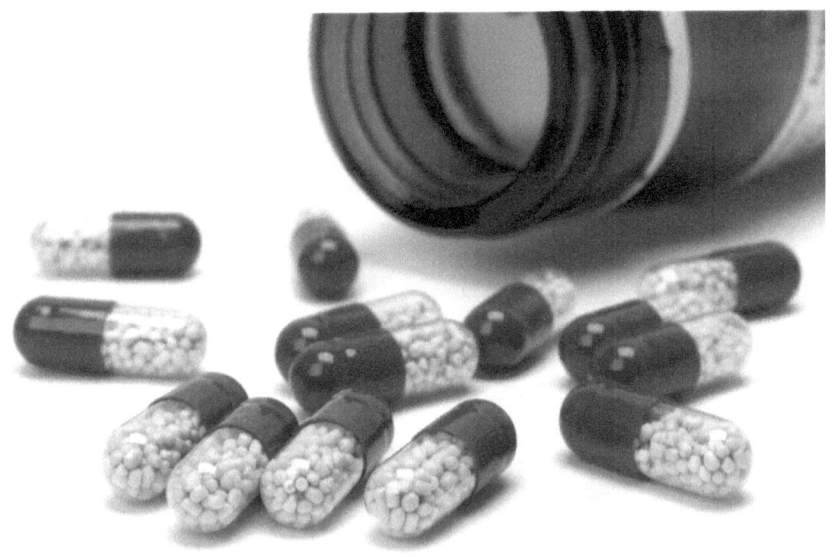

credits by freedigitalphotos.net

Benefits of Exercise

There are many different styles of exercise. My definition of exercise is any physical activity and movement that is responsible for promoting overall health. There are several ways to achieve a daily physical regiment such as, walking, running, dancing, mowing the lawn, gardening, and many other activities. Experts consider exercise that causes extreme discomfort or pain unhealthy with the potential to cause permanent damage to our bodies. Exercise can improve mood swings and mild depression because it helps you feel better on the inside and out. It is an amazing activity to boost one's self-esteem and give you an empowerment that cant be explained. A combination of nutrition and exercise will lead to a successful healthy weight loss because you will experience fat loss as well as increase muscle strength and a very welcomed increase in energy for the most part. There are so many benefits of exercise I could have really only written an exercise book. Because I have had more of the weight loss through diets instead of exercise, I didnt realize the importance of workout to a weight loss program. Nutrition and exercise work like a hand and a glove; the hand needs the glove to keep it warm. Exercise increases enzymes, which burn fat and increase metabolic rates to improve digestion. Exercise releases hormones called endorphins, which improve mood swings and depressions. Exercising on a regular basis in combination with a healthy diet can lower blood pressure and cholesterol to decrease your chances of heart attack and stroke. Weight bearing exercises are great for patients with osteoporosis because the exercises help build bone tissue. Breast cancer tumor production is linked to two hormones, which are estradiol and progesterone; these hormones are lowered by exercise.

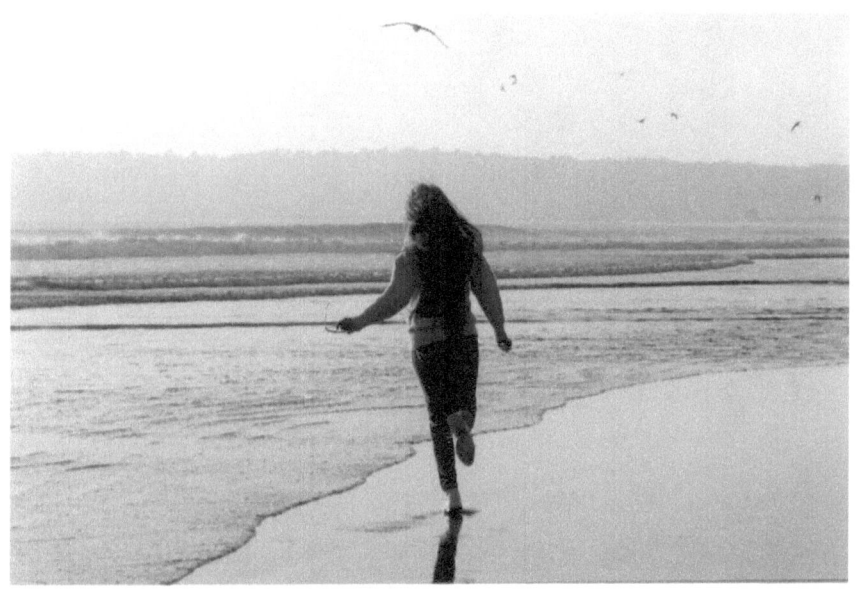

credits by freedigitalphotos.net

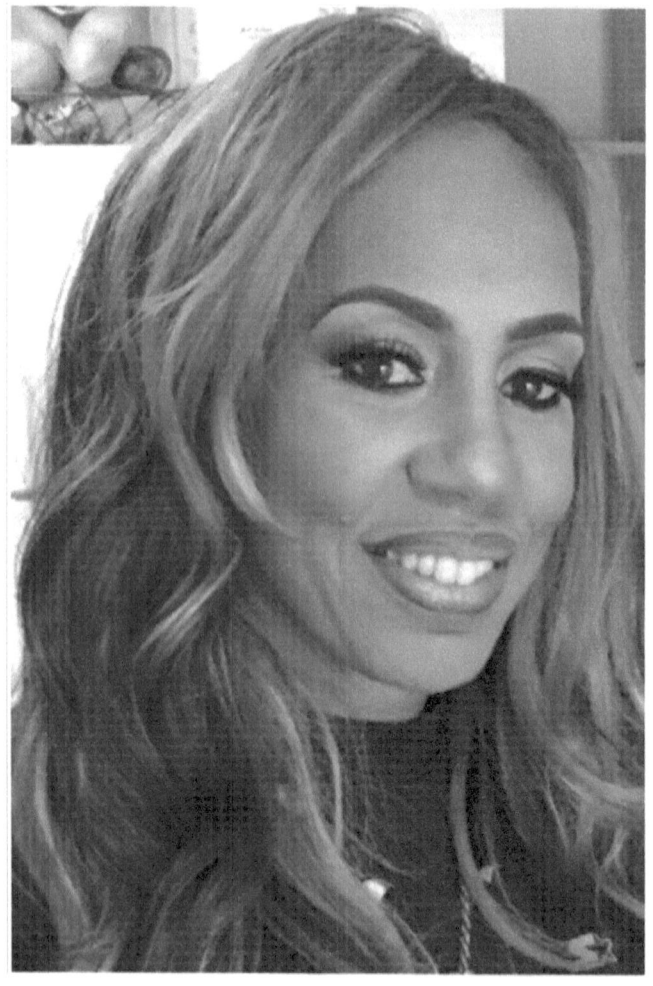

Remember when starting a new healthy weight loss program that includes Nutrition and Exercise it has to be something that you want for yourself.

You have to get motivated and stay motivated because the weight gain didn't occur overnight and it is not going to come off overnight either. The weight will come off with hard work and dedication. You remember when you were in your late teens to twenties? You could eat anything in sight and drink as much as you wanted. Your body was very forgiving and seemed to bounce back from any food and drink consumption. When you look around now, the predominant of people in their late thirties to early forties are dropping dead and having heart attacks because they become comfortable with lifestyles and bad habits that eventually catch up with them. I just hate that it took me so long to discover the importance of exercise. The good news is that you can regain the feeling of being more youthful at any age.

When starting a program, remember that the cure for motivation is actually seeing the results from your lifestyle change. You may even experience a weight gain at first but your body will start to take a t urn and the numbers on the scale will go down, down, down. Because I initially gained weight I am not married to the scale. For me it is better to consider my measurements because I have to remember FAT WEIGHS HALF THAT OF MUSCLE. Ask yourself how bad you want a change and what are your reasons for the change. Your first month will be crucial for you to stick to your plan because your body will be going through an adjustment period. If you hang in there, the results will come quickly. Read success stories of others to see if they have experienced some of the same challenges that you have had and see how they have overcome their challenges. As I said, I know how fat feels.

Morning exercises jump start your day and wake up the

metabolism to start the process of burning fat. Find a workout that you like to do. I will tell you about mine in just a second. The gym is not for everyone. I was one that would not get a gym membership because I was afraid I would waste my money but there are so many other things to do at the gym to achieve a complete workout. If you make it fun, it wont seem like a chore or something that just has to be done but something you enjoy. I can truly say I look forward to workouts now. One of the biggest secrets is keeping a positive attitude. If you dont want to use a trainer but you think that you need guidance, there are thousands of DVD workouts out there. Just search until you find the one that works for you.

Now let's get back to me. On May 13 of 2009 I decided to try something different with the weight loss. I weighed in at the 170's but usually my weight would fluctuate. I didnt consider myself fat but I knew that I needed to bring my weight down a notch. My eating habits were not a problem but I continued to maintain the same weight. As a result I decided to try something different; I discovered running. My goal was to train as if I planned to run a 5K marathon; at least I would be in shape. Initially I went to the track every day. I remember the first day I started; I was walking to warm up then I started running to see how far I could go. I thought I was going to need some oxygen so I knew that I wasnt ready but I didnt let that stop me. It just motivated me to work harder and run a little further every day. It also helps when you have a person in your life that shares the same goals of being healthy. I know I do. Instead of going out on dates, I have running dates then go out to lunch and the body will burn it right up; in addition, the muscles will get refueled. You dont have to run to get results. You can walk at a nice pace but the name of the game is getting the heart rate up, which you can achieve with a nice pace of physical activity. You can buy a watch that tracks the heart rate for you. I look forward to running but I know that I need rest days to allow proper healing of my muscles. When building muscles, tiny tears are created in the muscle fibers because you work them beyond their regular capacity. That's why you are very sore after a hard workout. Your muscles add a little tissue at the sight of the tear repairing themselves on their own.

If you dont permit sufficient rest time to allow your muscles to heal, you could damage tendons, ligaments and muscles, which could lead to long lasting constant pain. It is important to listen to your body. I had to learn to listen to my body. In the beginning you will experience soreness just because your muscles are not accustomed to a physical regiment. That is why we stretch before and after physical activity. Stretching, which is often overlooked and even left out it, helps to increase flexibility, endurance and strength and help to prevent injury. Stretching helps to increase our range of motion, which is sometimes affected by physical activity, age and gender.

Stretching warms the muscles and prepares them for the hard work as well as protects them from sprains and strains. Stretching decreases muscle soreness after a workout. Yoga classes are very good for increasing flexibility. Remember I am only making suggestions. Please consult your physician before starting anything new.

Some days are better for me as far as my workout so I know that a lot of it is mental. There are some days my body is saying, "What are you doing to me?" After I get started, I feel so much better and there are days where I can just run, run, run. Most days I run up to two miles and more than that sometimes. When I look back, I never thought that I would be actually running. I literally didnt like working out but I knew that I had to learn to **love** it to get the results that I wanted. If I only changed my eating habits at this point, I would not achieve what I wanted to see. I had to work out too. I also joined the gym to have a place to go when it is really cold outside or raining; therefore, I am going to take advantage of the machines too. I can see my body transforming right before my eyes; in addition, my endurance level is getting longer and longer. To have successful weight loss and healthy life style management you need to have sensible goals and keep your expectations realistic. This gives you a better chance to make this a lifestyle change. Another important aspect of weight loss is the necessity to burn more calories than you take in.

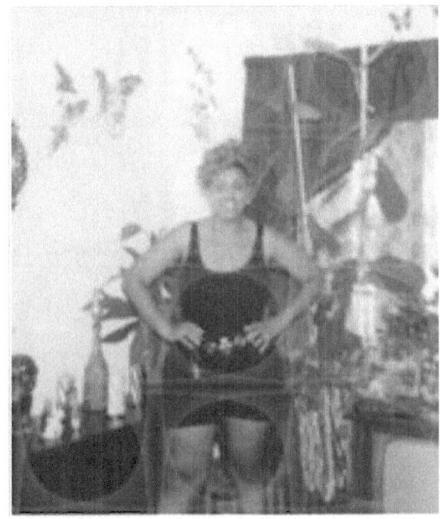

Before

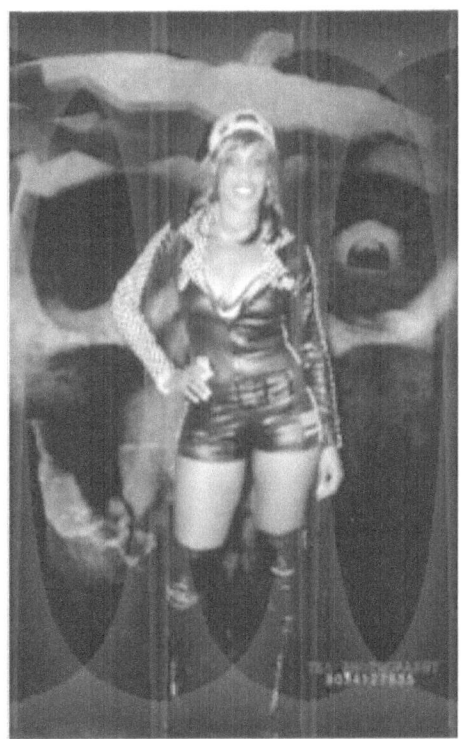

After

Conclusion

I pray and trust that I have touched many people with my experiences. Please believe me this will not be my last book. My next phase will go more in depth about the different topics that I have brought before you. If I had to give you advice, my first recommendation would encourage you to change your way of thinking. A diet has to be a healthy weight loss change. Ask God to help you make a commitment to the choices you have made to your new lifestyle. Replace negative thoughts with positive thoughts and avoid listening to feedback or criticism from people around you because they will tell you that you are losing too much weight. As a matter of fact according to the charts, I am still over weight but I am comfortable with the skin that I am in. Our bodies are designed to deviate from our regular regiment for a short period of time but before that happens you have to know when to say enough is enough and get back on a plan to eat right. Your body is your temple; you have to take care of it mentally, physically and spiritually to maintain feeling good on a daily basis.

When you change your way of life, things such as, self-confidence mysteriously appear. I have so much energy and I hold my head high. My level of confidence is out of this world. This is a good feeling. I used to hurt so badly and now I hurt for others that think a person has to be sick to lose weight. I realized that a person could actually step up, take control and make lifestyle changes. My weight was getting out of control so I knew that I needed to make a change for the better. Some days will be harder than others. Stay strong and write your feelings down. You have to find what works for you. I could give you a basic outline to go by but most people have to tweak it a little to fit their individual needs. As you educate yourself more and more the road to weight loss will get easier and easier. The foods that I once ate do not even taste the same because I have acquired a whole new taste for healthiness and the same will happen for you

Meal Plans

Everyday Healthy Living Food Chart

This chart has a list of realistic food choices to help you sustain a healthy lifestyle.

Meats:

Ground (sirloin)

Top Round

Recommend all types of seafood

Limit your shrimp if you have high cholesterol.

Try to eat fish 3 to 5 times weekly

(Pork) if you desire keep to a minimum same as beef lean cuts.

Beef (Very lean cuts limit 2 times weekly)

Remember it takes beef 3 days to digest in your system

Veal (round, chop, cutlets)

Chicken Turkey

Poultry:

Chicken

Turkey Breast

Ground turkey

Turkey bacon

Turkey sausage

Cornish Hen

Limit sandwich meat, when choosing sandwich meat it is

best that it is either low sodium, fat free or low fat.

Dairy:

Cheese (Fat free or 2%)
Swiss
American
Cheddar
Mozzarella
Parmesan
String
Cream and Cottage Cheese (fat free or low fat)
Eggs (use eggs, egg whites or eggs substitute)—served boiled poached, if you scramble your eggs use "Pam" cooking oil.
Milk—1% or 2% of fat free
Soymilk/ Soy protein—low fat
Yogurt (choose ones that are low fat or low carbohydrate count.)
Yogurt is good to replace good bacteria lining of the intestine and it helps to control Candida and yeast.

Nuts:

Peanuts (handful) 2 teaspoons of Peanut Butter
Pecans
Almonds Macadamias
Cashews
Pistachios-all nuts are limited to 20 pieces

Spices and Seasoning:

(No sugar added/ lemon juice)

Pepper

Garlic

Cayenne

Hot Sauce

Ms Dash

McCormick

Mustard

Low fat Mayo 2 teaspoons

Treats: (all sugar free)

Hard candy

Fudge icicles

Sugar Free Pudding

Gelatin

Gum

Pop icicles

Fruits: Any fruit is good

Examples:

Apples

Pears

Berries

Plums

Peaches

Grapes

Oranges

Limit bananas, which are high in sugar

(The more raw thebetter)

Vegetables:

(The more raw veggies the better)

Legumes

Lettuce (all kinds) free food-meaning you can eat as much as you want.

Cucumbers—no limit

Broccoli-no limit Spinach-no limit

Celery-no limit

Mushrooms-all kinds

Tomatoes (Dont eat with beef you could retain fluid in your body.)

Greens-all sort

Cabbage

Cauliflower

Squash-no limit

Alfalfa

Zucchini

Onions

All peppers—green, yellow, orange, red

Carrots (high in Glycemic Index Fat)

Vegetable (Canola/ Olive Oils)—You can use Pam cooking Sprays.

Breads: (sparingly)

High fiber, low carbohydrate, wheat breads—2 slices
Pita bread ½, Whole grain bagel ½
Oat & Rye Bread (Melba Toast 2 with meal)
Low fat-High fiber tortillas

Cereal (All high fibers 3 grams and up)
Special K
Fiber One
Extra Fiber—All bran
(Make sure all cereal is high in fiber and low in sugar.)

Pasta (Whole wheat; limit to once per week)
Potato ½ Baked or Sweet (don't have bread with it.)—High in potassium.
Brown Rice-1 cup (sparingly)

Your day should consist of:

1. Breakfast
2. Midday morning snack
3. Lunch
4. After lunch snack
5. Dinner
6. Evening snack

~Try to exercise 3 to 5 days a week for 30 minutes and up ~

Sample Meal:

- Breakfast—½ grapefruit, scrambled egg with 2 slices of turkey bacon, Decaf coffee or tea with nonfat milk and add a sugar substitute (example Splenda or equal.)

- Midday Snack—4 oz low fat yogurt

- Lunch—Tuna salad with onions, tomatoes, 1 tablespoon of mayonnaise, in whole-wheat pita bread.

- After Lunch Snack—1 small red apple

- Dinner-Grilled chicken breast with green peppers and onions over 1 cup of brown rice, table salad topped with low fat dressing.

- Evening Snack-15 Almonds

*For the first three days we are going to do *"Let's get it Started"*. That is when we eat protein and veggies for the first 3 days, excluding any complex carbohydrates and desserts sugar free/ fat free fudge icicles at that time.

A sample of "Let's get it Started" is:

- Breakfast—Egg beaters add any veggies you like (creating an omelet) with turkey sausage or two strips of turkey bacon.

- Mid Snack—Veggie sticks of your choice: carrots, broccoli, celery sticks w/ low fat dressing.

- Lunch-1 chicken breast, veggies of your choice or a big salad, (sugar free dessert.)

- Dinner—Broiled fish bowl and cooked or raw Veggies

- During the "Let's Get Started" phase you should experience weight loss this helps to get metabolism elevated.

- You should drink at least 2 liters of water a day (no concentrated fruit juices.) Limit diet soda to 2 a day, clear flavored water, crystal light.

- Subway has a really good salad selection ("I eat one just every day.")

- I really dont want to start measuring your foods just remember that your meat size should be about the size of the inside of your hand.

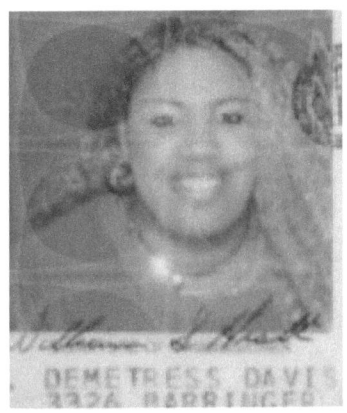

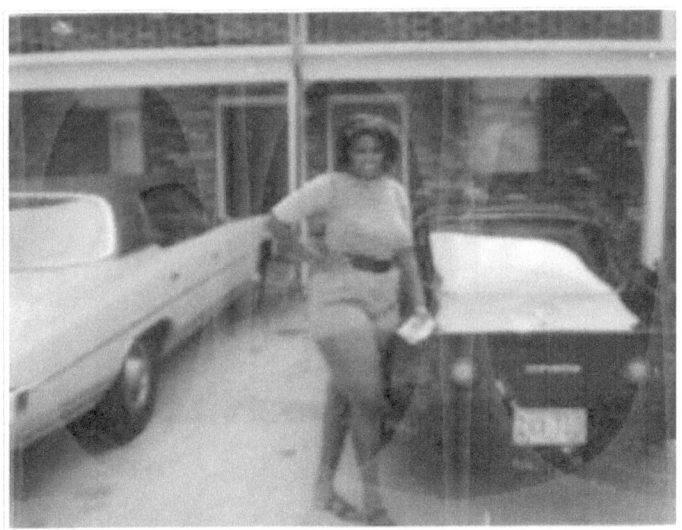

Meal Journals with Recorded Emotions

Date:

Breakfast:

_____

_____

AM Snack:

_____

_____

Lunch:

_____

_____

Afternoon Snack:

_____

_____

Dinner:

_____

_____

EMOTIONS:

_____

_____

Date:

Breakfast:

_____

_____

AM Snack:

_____

_____

Lunch:

_____

_____

Afternoon Snack:

_____

_____

Dinner:

_____

_____

EMOTIONS:

_____

_____

Date:

Breakfast:

_____

_____

AM Snack:

_____

_____

Lunch:

_____

_____

Afternoon Snack:

_____

_____

Dinner:

_____

_____

EMOTIONS:

_____

_____

Date:

Breakfast:

_____

_____

AM Snack:

_____

_____

Lunch:

_____

_____

Afternoon Snack:

_____

_____

Dinner:

_____

_____

EMOTIONS:

_____

_____

Date:

Breakfast:

_____

_____

AM Snack:

_____

_____

Lunch:

_____

_____

Afternoon Snack:

_____

_____

Dinner:

_____

_____

EMOTIONS:

_____

_____

Date:

Breakfast:

_____

_____

AM Snack:

_____

_____

Lunch:

_____

_____

Afternoon Snack:

_____

_____

Dinner:

_____

_____

EMOTIONS:

_____

_____

Date:

Breakfast:

_____

_____

AM Snack:

_____

_____

Lunch:

_____

_____

Afternoon Snack:

_____

_____

Dinner:

_____

_____

EMOTIONS:

_____

_____

Date:

Breakfast:

_____

_____

AM Snack:

_____

_____

Lunch:

_____

_____

Afternoon Snack:

_____

_____

Dinner:

_____

_____

EMOTIONS:

_____

_____

Date:

Breakfast:

_____

_____

AM Snack:

_____

_____

Lunch:

_____

_____

Afternoon Snack:

_____

_____

Dinner:

_____

_____

EMOTIONS:

_____

_____

Date:

Breakfast:

_____

_____

AM Snack:

_____

_____

Lunch:

_____

_____

Afternoon Snack:

_____

_____

Dinner:

_____

_____

EMOTIONS:

_____

_____

Date:

Breakfast:

_____

_____

AM Snack:

_____

_____

Lunch:

_____

_____

Afternoon Snack:

_____

_____

Dinner:

_____

_____

EMOTIONS:

_____

_____

Date:

Breakfast:

_____

_____

AM Snack:

_____

_____

Lunch:

_____

_____

Afternoon Snack:

_____

_____

Dinner:

_____

_____

EMOTIONS:

_____

_____

Date:

Breakfast:

_____

_____

AM Snack:

_____

_____

Lunch:

_____

_____

Afternoon Snack:

_____

_____

Dinner:

_____

_____

EMOTIONS:

_____

_____

Date:

Breakfast:

_____

_____

AM Snack:

_____

_____

Lunch:

_____

_____

Afternoon Snack:

_____

_____

Dinner:

_____

_____

EMOTIONS:

_____

_____

Date:

Breakfast:

_____

_____

AM Snack:

_____

_____

Lunch:

_____

_____

Afternoon Snack:

_____

_____

Dinner:

_____

_____

EMOTIONS:

_____

_____

Date:

Breakfast:

_____

_____

AM Snack:

_____

_____

Lunch:

_____

_____

Afternoon Snack:

_____

_____

Dinner:

_____

_____

EMOTIONS:

_____

_____

Date:

Breakfast:

_____

_____

AM Snack:

_____

_____

Lunch:

_____

_____

Afternoon Snack:

_____

_____

Dinner:

_____

_____

EMOTIONS:

_____

_____

Date:

Breakfast:

_____

_____

AM Snack:

_____

_____

Lunch:

_____

_____

Afternoon Snack:

_____

_____

Dinner:

_____

_____

EMOTIONS:

_____

_____

Date:

Breakfast:

_____

_____

AM Snack:

_____

_____

Lunch:

_____

_____

Afternoon Snack:

_____

_____

Dinner:

_____

_____

EMOTIONS:

_____

_____

Date:

Breakfast:

_____

_____

AM Snack:

_____

_____

Lunch:

_____

_____

Afternoon Snack:

_____

_____

Dinner:

_____

_____

EMOTIONS:

_____

_____